My Gift To You

iUniverse, Inc.
New York Bloomington

My Gift to You
Encouragement During a Cancer Crisis

Copyright © 2009 by Ruth Olson

Unless otherwise noted, all Scripture quotations are taken from the New International Version of the Bible.

iUniverse books may be ordered through booksellers or by contacting:

iUniverse
1663 Liberty Drive
Bloomington, IN 47403
www.iuniverse.com
1-800-Authors (1-800-288-4677)

ISBN: 978-1-4401-4574-2 (pbk)
ISBN: 978-1-4401-4575-9(ebk)

Printed in the United States of America

Library of Congress Control Number: 2009930577

iUniverse rev. date: 6/26/2009

My Gift To You

Encouragement During A Cancer Crisis

Ruth Olson

Dedication

This book is dedicated to my husband, Jerry, who provided the love I so needed to make it through to victory. Thanks, honey.

Foreword

About a half-century ago, my Christian college physiology professor predicted that by the beginning of the 21st century, a cure for cancer would have been found. Instead, he said, most of us would die from heart problems, for die we all would. Yet, he reminded us: We do not live to ourselves, and we do not die to ourselves. If we live, we live to the Lord, and if we die, we die to the Lord; so then, whether we live or whether we die, we are the Lord's. (Romans 14:7-8 NRSV)

The year 2000 has come and gone. And so has this professor's prediction.

Today we know that everyone has at least a few cancer cells. For nearly two-thirds of us, our natural defenses will keep cancer from taking hold. My sister, Ruth, is one of the one-third for whom this wasn't true. On these pages she reaches out to you—a cancer patient, relative, or friend—with words to deal with this deadly disease. She writes honestly, but also lovingly, for Ruth has lived "to the Lord" all of her life.

She wrote these pages for one reason only—to help you.

Ruth also lives in God's hope. God's love and promises sustained her throughout her healing. May they also strengthen and comfort you.

May the God of hope fill you with all joy and peace in

believing, so that you may abound in hope by the power of the Holy Spirit. (Romans 15:13 NRSV)

Alice Stolper Peppler
Author of *Divorced: Surviving the Pain*
Alice 'n Ink Editing
apeppler@aol.com

A Note From The Author

Dear Reader,

I had no intention of writing about my experience with cancer. With endless numbers of books on the subject, the thought never occurred to me that one more would add anything of value.

I had begun to write on another subject when I veered in the direction of the book you're now holding. Throughout my cancer experience, I realized that there were things regarding my journey, though difficult at times that needed to be addressed.

I have never had anyone ask outright what it is like to have cancer, but perhaps you have wondered silently and have questions. Neither have I had anyone near and dear to me suffer with cancer. But maybe you have, and are now searching for answers in dealing with your stricken loved one. Nor have I dealt with the needs of a neighbor with cancer, but perhaps the woman next door may have just confided in you a doctor's diagnosis of her cancer.

And, just maybe, you yourself are a cancer victim.

I fortunately have never laid a loved one to rest after a cancer struggle, but you perhaps have. If so, my prayers are with you.

I never thought I would get cancer, but I did. I agonized if I would survive, and I did. This book may hold some answers to your questions. I hope so, because it's *my gift to you.* –Ruth Olson

Contents

Chapter One

Fear of the Unknown

"When you come to the end of all the light you know, and it's time to step into the darkness of the unknown, faith is knowing that one of two things will happen: either you will be given something solid to stand on or you will be taught to fly."
-Edward Teller

My story began in a fall season before the colorful leaves started dropping from the trees. I was quite content with life, but unbeknown to me a crisis was on the horizon raising its repulsive head; growing ever so slowly perhaps invading my body I was told up to one and one half years prior.

Not until months later, in February 2004, was I diagnosed with breast cancer.

Doctors called it a "big, ugly" breast cancer. There were three separate tumors, diagnosed as invasive ductal carcinoma. I barely comprehended its judgment call when pronounced. The memories now grab me, forcing me to remember.

Looking back, I realize I've always had in me a subconscious fear of cancer. A generalized dread of it hung overhead, as an ominous cloud covering my universe. I felt a chill each time the subject of cancer was in the news, or when a commercial reminded me my annual mammogram was due, or when I heard that a friend had been stricken with cancer. It loomed its ugly, revolting head again and again. It was omnipresent to be sure, but certainly not yet personal. I would often pray for those with breast cancer with the assurance that I would never get it. At least that is what I told myself.

Then out from the darkness the lightening struck! Its blow was hard—a direct hit to my heart! It knocked me out of my zone of solitude and contentment into one of fear and confusion!

Diagnosed with a disease such as cancer is shocking at the very least. I could hardly comprehend the magnitude of it all. My thoughts became mangled. In many sufferers anger, denial, defeat, depression, to name a few possible reactions, can appear suddenly. But one of the feelings that stands out is fear. Fear of the unknown can be debilitating.

I wondered what would happen to me. Where would this dreaded disease take me? Slipping into the unknown, I barely noticed where I was headed. My thoughts tumbled over one another; my faith in God flip-flopped. Would I be healed? First I was certain, but then unsure. I was drowning in a mystery of words spoken by those in control now of my body and senses.

Who were these people who suddenly invaded my space? Their instructions included directions of when to come and go; to lie still, to listen, to comprehend what now was so important. I'd hear, "You'll be carefully watched and monitored." "Your surgery is scheduled after chemotherapy." "Radiation follows after more chemotherapy." "Take these medications." "Be here at this time." And the terminology was completely new to me. It was as if I was suddenly forced to learn an entire new language on a moment's notice. Being a retired R.N. didn't apply in this situation. I just couldn't wrap my thoughts around what was happening to me, personally or professionally. It was surreal.

It is not every day one is challenged by death. To realize that it has your name with no intention of ever relinquishing its hold is sobering. One cannot shake off all too quickly the thoughts of death.

In past circumstances I had used this verse in claiming peace for others at the death of loved ones, "Where, O death, is your victory? Where, O death, is your sting?" (I Corinthians 15:55). In a following verse, 57, it reads: "But thanks be to God! He gives us the victory through our Lord Jesus Christ."

Without a doubt, in Christ we have the victory over death, and seeing death from afar I was safe and secure in my faith. However, now it was I who was feeling the sting; death suddenly became real to me and certainly a possibility. The Lord was pulling me through the eye of the needle of death. In my spirit I knew it, and physically, I could do nothing about it. To cope, I went into denial. I laughed it off, often making light of the subject. To many I quipped, "If it is as bad as they say, why haven't I died?" I remember distinctly the silent reaction to that statement of mine.

I certainly hoped I would be all right. However, I had yet to "feel" anything—I had no physical pain whatsoever. I could hardly comprehend that I was even sick, let alone diagnosed with cancer. Nevertheless, if the diagnosis was accurate I told myself I would trust in the Lord.

In Psalm 31:13-15, David said, "There is terror on every side. . . But I trust in you, O Lord; I say, you are my God. My times are in thy hand. . . ."

Some Advice

When fear shows itself in forms such as doubt and anger, deal with it through your personal faith in the Lord Jesus Christ. During your initial time of planning your treatment and cure with your mate, family, and medical team, keep your faith focused on Him, the author and perfecter of your faith. "Let us fix our eyes on Jesus, the author and perfecter of our faith, who for the joy set before him endured the cross, scorning its shame, and sat down at the right hand of the throne of God." (Hebrews 12:2) God will not fail you or desert you. Nothing in all creation is hidden from His sight; He knows what is going on in your life right now. Saturate your mind with the Word of God. Proverbs 3:1 reads, "My son, do not forget my teaching, but keep my commands in your heart, for they will prolong your life many years and bring you prosperity."

Use this opportunity to memorize Scripture; those verses you always have wanted to but never seemed to have the time. Let your doctors keep track of your medications and treatments and you keep track of your faith level. Place your fears in the Lord's hands. He will restore your faith and take you under His wings of healing. "But for you who revere my name, the sun of righteousness will rise with healing in its wings. And you will go out and leap like calves released from the stall." (Malachi 4:2)

". . . do not fear, for I am with you; do not be dismayed, for I am your God. I will strengthen you and help you; I will uphold you with my righteous right hand." (Isaiah 41:10).

"The Lord is my light and my salvation—whom shall I fear? The Lord is the stronghold of my life—of whom shall I be afraid?" (Psalm 27:1)

Let's pray together:

Dear Father,

Everything I'm going through right now brings a shadow of fear on me and my family causing great concern and worries. Please shine your light into my darkness. Show me a way where there seems to be none. Help me to trust in you with all this change in my body, mind and spirit. Guide the medical team and my loved ones as they reach out to me. Lord, your love gives me courage. I rest in you. In Jesus' name. Amen.

Chapter Two

Doubts Dispersed

"The Lord is near to all who call upon Him."
(Psalm 145:18)

"Ruth, you have my admiration—how you deal with all your adversaries and are looking forward to victory." (Hannelore, Wisconsin)

I received many notes similar to the above one in regards to my cancer diagnosis. Each one I opened touched me and showed how caring people in the body of Christ are when they reach out to one another in love.

There was another helpful person who totally changed my attitude when the doctors first disclosed my diagnosis. The impact of that diagnosis of cancer was not only devastating to me, but also to those who were near and dear to me. We were all baffled and taken aback after hearing the unexpected news. As mentioned, I found myself in denial; my loved ones were silent. I didn't know exactly how to go about entering this endless sphere of questions on my part and neither did those about me.

Thankfully, a young doctor came to my rescue. His simple solution to my bewilderment supplied a foundation of strength and direction guiding me to next step. I found myself in his office for some reason, now forgotten, and just as he was leaving, I suddenly blurted out the diagnosis of cancer pinned on me, and asked him what he thought. I barely knew the man, but I felt I was to ask of him what I couldn't supply myself to calm my mind and heart. Little did I know the Lord would use his comments to my advantage throughout my entire ordeal.

With a thoughtful look on his face he turned around, releasing his hand from the doorknob. I was grateful he was willing to take the time to explore this added concern of mine.

"This is not my area of expertise," he pondered, "and I only comment because my mother had breast cancer, but I have learned this much: each person's case is different; each diagnosis is different, and each treatment and recovery is different. Never compare your situation with another's," he emphasized.

With that, he turned around and left. I was immediately shoved into reality with his God-given words. Oh, how they lifted me up over the threshold and through the door of the unknown.

This truth he spoke laid out a path for me to take. With it as a banner above me, I proceeded to walk forward confident the Lord was indeed with me and would guide me accordingly in each season of the disease. I was unique and my situation *was* different from others! I could trust the Lord to lead me in dealing with doctors, medication, treatment, bad days along with good days, and ultimately peace of mind.

Scripture says, "If any of you lacks wisdom, he should ask God, who gives generously to all without finding fault, and it will be given to him. But when he asks, he must believe and not doubt, because he who doubts is like a wave of the sea, blown and tossed by the wind." (James 1:5, 6) Without the revelation from this doctor, I was like a wave of the sea blown and tossed by the wind. Thankfully, my doubts no longer existed. The Lord took my fears away.

Grounded in His Love

"Come to me, all you who are weary and burdened, and I will give you rest." (Matthew 11:28)

You, too, may need grounding, first in the assurance that there are loved ones and friends who are supporting you, along with a medical team who is working with you planning the course to receive the best medical treatment. But also, the necessity of building up your faith in Christ Jesus is imperative now. Again, a verse that helped me during this time was Psalm 32:7, "You are my hiding place; you will protect me from trouble and surround me with songs of deliverance."

Being grounded in the Word of God gives you the underlying strength needed to continue even if the path gets difficult or takes an unexpected turn. By digging your roots deep into the Word of God it gives you reassurance that you are grounded in faith and hope in Him.

Here are some verses to help you through the hard times in any crisis:

"Even though I walk through the valley of the shadow of death, I will fear no evil, for you are with me; your rod and your staff, they comfort me."(Psalm 23:4)

"Praise the Lord, O my soul, and forget not all his

benefits—who forgives all your sins and heals all your diseases." (Psalm 103:2, 3)

"But he was pierced for our transgressions, he was crushed for our iniquities; the punishment that brought us peace was upon him, and by his wounds we are healed." (Isaiah 53:5)

". . . (He) healed all the sick." (Matthew 8:16b)

"This was to fulfill what was spoken through the prophet Isaiah: 'He took up our infirmities and carried our diseases.'" (Matthew 8:17)

". . . pay attention to what I say; listen close to my words. Do not let them out of your sight, keep them within your heart; for they are life to those who find them and health to a man's whole body." (Proverbs 4:20-22)

"If you remain in me and my words remain in you, ask whatever you wish, and it will be given you." (John 15:7)

"But those who suffer he delivers in their suffering; he speaks to them in their affliction." (Job 36:15)

"For the Lord God is a sun and shield; the Lord bestows favor and honor; no good thing does he withhold from those whose walk is blameless." (Psalm 84:11)

"Jesus went throughout Galilee, teaching in their

synagogues, preaching the good news for the kingdom, and healing every disease and sickness among the people." *(*Matthew 4:23)

"Call upon me in the day of trouble; I will deliver you, and you will honor me." (Psalm 50:15)

"And the prayer offered in faith will make the sick person well; the Lord will raise him up. If he has sinned, he will be forgiven." (James 5:15)

Let's pray together:

Dear Father God, I am sick. I am suffering. My physical condition is weighing heavily on me and my family. I am surrounded by distractions and my mind drifts at times from your precious Word. Please give me peace of mind and peace of heart. Take me in your loving arms and surround me with your mercy and healing. May your love give me strength to continue this walk. In Jesus name. Amen.

Chapter Three

God Does Love Us

"The depth of our faith is not to be judged by how much we have received, but rather by how long we can wait and receive nothing."
-Author unknown

Why must we experience pain? Why discomfort? Why suffering? I remember asking God, "Why me, Lord?" I believe His silent reply in my heart was, "Why not you, Ruth?"

God has a plan for all of us and that often includes suffering this side of Heaven. There are a few afflicted souls who just refuse to go through the pain and suffering part of discipleship. "It's too hard." "This must be of Satan." "I know I just can't make it." "I've had enough!" A thought-provoking quote from Madame Jeanne Guyon, (1648-1717) the French mystic, is: "If knowing answers to life's questions is absolutely necessary to you, then forget the journey. You will never make it, for this is a journey of unknowables--of unanswered questions, enigmas, incomprehensibles, and most of all, things unfair."

Trials can seem unfair, but God promises us worthwhile results by going through an upheaval in our lifetime. This is shown in Romans 5:3, "...we also rejoice in our sufferings, because we know that suffering produces perseverance; perseverance, character; and character, hope. And hope does not disappoint us, because God has poured out his love into our hearts by the Holy Spirit, whom he has given us." II Corinthians 4:17 says something similar: "For our light and momentary troubles are achieving for us an eternal glory that far outweighs them all. So we fix our eyes not on what is seen, but on what is unseen. For what is seen is temporary, but what is unseen is eternal."

Obedience in suffering does have its compensation: it produces a lasting fruit providing we do not give up on God having His perfect way in us. Through our trials, God breaks our strong will and sinful mindset. Romans 8:5 speaks of this mindset: "Those who live according to the sinful nature have their minds set on what that nature desires…" This is a mindset of "self," of "getting our way," of having a pity party," and having a "Why is this happening to me?" attitude.

I came across a quote years ago and it may apply here: "All people regard all change as loss and it is followed by anger." We can't always predict the changes in our life; some are harsh and cruel and can appear as resulting in a loss to us. Anger may follow when we don't get our way, when the change, as in the case of not being healed, is a huge inconvenience to us. Our rights have been violated, or so we feel, and we get angry at God, at man, and at ourselves.

It's during these times that suffering, trials, or pain are allowed by God in His perfect design to move us away from self and move us closer to Him. Dawn Spurlin who suffered from cancer in 2005, said, "I learned that the reason I am suffering is not that God wanted to punish me, but because He wanted to draw me closer." ("How

Would You Respond to Cancer?" from Voice in the Wilderness, July 2005, Vol: 12, Issue 7.)

When we finally accept what the Lord has for us, including all discomforts and demanding detours in our lives, we receive the peace of mind in Christ Jesus. Granted, we may not be healed immediately, or the problem may never disappear, but we will be brought in a place of acknowledging, "Not my will, but yours, O Lord."

And there are other causes of suffering. The result of our trials often leads to the glory of God. Remember the story of Joseph whose brothers sold him into slavery? (See Genesis 37-50.) After suffering from a false accusation at the hand of his slave master's wife, Joseph landed in prison. Because the Lord used him to interpret the Cupbearer and the Baker's dreams and later the Pharaoh's, he was vindicated and placed in a position second-in-command under Pharaoh. When his brothers came to Egypt for food to survive a great famine, Joseph recognized them and eventually had them send for their father, Jacob. The family remained in Egypt throughout the famine. Then Jacob died. Joseph's brothers, thinking that he would have them put to death for what they had done by selling him into slavery, fell at this feet and begged for mercy. Joseph said these reassuring words to his brothers, "Don't be afraid. Am I in the place of God? You intended to harm me, but God intended it for good to accomplish what is not being done, the saving of many lives." (Genesis 50:19) God's plan for our lives often times is unknown to us, but by faith we are encouraged to believe that whatever we are going through, there is a godly reason for it.

Sickness unto Death

And then there is a sickness unto death. Dear friend, if your loved one has died due to a sickness, be aware that the Lord knows your grief. One of my favorite verses regarding death is Isaiah 57:1 (TLB): "The good men perish; the godly die before their time and no one seems to care or wonder why. No one seems to realize that God is taking them away from evil days ahead. For the godly who die shall rest in peace." You can receive comfort from the words of Scripture.

I mention in my book, *Jesus Loves You This I Know*, (Page 98, ACW Press), God listens to the person's heart as death nears. "Remember the thief on the cross with Jesus? Read the account in Luke 23:32-43. There were two thieves crucified with Jesus. One denied Christ with his dying words. The other realized his own sin and acknowledged the Son of God. With his dying breath, the repentant thief asked Jesus to remember him, and Jesus answered, 'I tell you the truth, today you will be with me in paradise.' We have no way of knowing if this thief even knew of Jesus before this moment. What we do know is recorded: Jesus heard this thief's cry for mercy and acted on it."

God loves us and meets us where there is no other answer to our situation.

Let's pray together:

Dear Father,

My trial is heavy on me. Please show me your faithfulness through my burden of _____. (Add your trial, such as sickness, loneliness, emotional pain, financial crisis, etc.) I know you love me. Make me aware of your love as we walk hand in hand each day toward victory. In Jesus' name. Amen.

Chapter Four

The Presence of Jesus

"When life caves in, you do not need reasons—you need comfort. You do not need some answers—you need someone. And Jesus does not come to us with an explanation—He comes to us with His presence."
-Bob Benson

During my cancer treatments, I received letters from many who were going through their own battle, or who had pushed through to victory. These following letters are from those who wanted to share their experiences to encourage others. The letters show how our Lord's presence is real.

The following letter is from Sue of Wisconsin suffering from cancer:

> Since March, 2006, I have experienced incredible kindness from people and a season of such tender love from our Lord. I was diagnosed with lung cancer, and all of life was put on hold during the chemo treatments. Work stopped all the running around stopped. Just the essentials remained--the Lord Jesus, His Word, my dear family, and some very dear Christian friends. My heart was touched and I was taught things that have changed me

forever. I literally felt carried through this time. During my CAT scan, I felt such tenderness from the Lord, as though He was preparing me and setting me down in a wide, grassy field, with a kiss on the top of my head, and saying to me, "Be strong. Be well."

A summary of another letter this one from Lois, which follows, came when I was first diagnosed with cancer. The amazing story of this woman, and another lady the Lord used, convinced me to consider getting a second opinion regarding my diagnosis of breast cancer. The marvel of this was that neither lady knew the other, but each was obedient to the Holy Spirit promptings to contact me after reading *Gentle Doves*. (A publication sent out bi-monthly by Ruth Olson Ministries.) Unbeknown to each, they both recommended the *same* clinic where I eventually transferred to for treatment resulting in a full recovery.

A summary of a letter from Lois:

Lois was diagnosed with breast cancer over eight years ago, and at the time she had a lumpectomy followed by radiation. In 2004 she had discomfort on the affected side and upon returning to the same clinic/hospital, tests showed "metastasis to the left humerus, left hip, right breastbone, and spot on her lung and four spots in her liver." As a result the doctor and nurse met her in the office and she said they "gave me a hug and walked out after saying, 'we're so sorry,' adding that she take an estrogen inhibitor and return in two years." Instead, Lois decided to contact another clinic, the one recommended to me by her and another woman, whereupon she received immediate treatment to curtail the cancer.

Always consider getting a second opinion. Take a leap of faith, and trust God to lead you accordingly. He doesn't lead us down a dead-end alley. You may have heard of the saying, "God is the 11 o'clock Lord." It suggests that our Lord sometimes comes in at the last minute with an answer. I asked the Lord to make it perfectly clear if He wanted me to contact another cancer clinic. I had one week before my scheduled mastectomy, and I had to act fast if I was to go elsewhere for treatment. He answered that prayer by getting me in to see the head doctor of the referred clinic, just days before my surgery. From that point on, the Lord healed me in record time through the treatment and love given me. Remember He is that near to you while you go through your trial, giving you counsel in your decisions.

Joyce of Minnesota writes about her pastor husband diagnosed with advanced gastric cancer. After his abdominal surgery, Joyce pens,

> I knew nothing would ever be the same.
> I was unraveled and my compass was
> missing. Over the months to follow, my
> husband lived a fairly normal life for
> which we thanked God. Suddenly every-
> thing reversed and hospice was signed on

for five months prior to the Lord taking him home.

In my memory, I returned to the view from my living room of the woods. I noticed the limbs of all the empty-browns were lifted upward toward the sky—every limb—and in the midst of them, a tall and perfect paper-white Birch tree. The one white tree in the midst of bleakness caused me to remember Jesus Christ, who stood alone for us in the midst of a crisis unlike any we could know. No one lifted arms to praise Him, and the cross He bore was splintered and certainly empty-brown. I knew that in Christ's season was my solution for my tears, emotions, confusion, future world of change, and for however long a time it took for me to walk through my woods. I made a decision to praise God, knowing and believing His promises. My husband and I praised God together. Now he is with Jesus 24-7, praising Him. God's plan for our lives included this hardship. Without Christ my thoughts would rationalize answers, and my emotions would flounder like the sea. I would only be seeking simple band aids to care for the enormous obstacle that seemed at that moment impossible. No amount of friends, activities, money or travel would bring me out of the woods. Winter's bleakness and browns do come. Crying is a refreshing fountain. There is an answer to the inevitable feelings of dead- ended despair that formulate the question, "How will I make it?" I believe a tree always plays a striking part in every loss and crisis. At first it might be burdensome, thorny, and empty-brown. Jesus is the pure white to gaze on amidst all empty-browns. But He is much more. He has won victory over the power of death and the fear of death.I Peter 2:24 is a verse we coveted, "He bore our sins on the Tree—by whose stripes we are healed." Empty-browns do not last forever. Remember birds rest in *ever*-greens from which victorious crosses are hewn. . . and rejoice!

The following testimony is from Fran from Wisconsin. She writes:

My cancer was rated between 3 and 4, the number 4 is considered terminal. I was in trouble. From the very beginning, the worst thing was NOT the cancer, it was the fear. To overcome fear was the biggest fight I had. After the initial biopsy and diagnosis of the cancerous lump on my neck, I remember waking up one night and feeling like I was being strangled. In the place where the lump had been removed, a second and bigger lump was there. My husband was led to pray Psalm

31 and Psalm 94. The next morning, it was gone. The doctor couldn't explain it. The doctors wanted to do a test on my hip that was supposed to be very painful and I had to be awake for it. When the day came, friends and relatives stayed outside my room and prayed in tongues; the staff didn't know what to think of it. I was told repeatedly that the procedure would be very painful, but I was asked to sign permission for them to do the other hip too. Most patients refuse to sign because of such terrible pain. My sister had called and told me that the Lord woke her up in the night and told her that everything would be all right. I signed the sheet. There was absolutely no pain with either hip procedure, and I had to have the test repeated with both hips, but still no pain.

I learned something about doctors that day. They won't own to anything different than what they think are ironclad facts. They don't usually acknowledge a miracle. The doctor's only explanation that the tests weren't painful for me was that some tolerate pain more than others. I was then scheduled for an exploratory operation that would remove the lymph nodes and my spleen and part of my liver. In the meantime, my church was praying and fasting for me. I told the doctor the cancer was going away. Every night I put my hands on the spot and told the cancer to shrink in the name of Jesus. It appeared more real to me every time I prayed. It was recommended surgery and I gave in. I shouldn't have. There was no cancer found. Afterwards, I started radiation treatment followed with chemotherapy. I didn't get sick with either. I continued to believe I was healed and visualized the cancer melting away. Since 1989 they haven't found any cancer. I give God all the glory! Hallelujah!

Notice how you can open your heart to the Lord's peace and healing by just giving over to Him the dilemma you find yourself in? He is always there for you. His presence is in each of these letters, all in different ways as the writer recalls the experience. "Cast all your anxiety on him because he cares for you." (I Peter 5:7)

Let's Pray Together:

Thank you, Lord Jesus, for all you've done,
Thank you, Lord.
Thank you, Jesus, for victories won,
Thank you, Lord.
For your love,
For your word and answered prayer,
Thank you, Jesus, for all you've done.
Thank you, Lord.

From an old hymn

Chapter Five

Thank God for Kindness

"In the compassion of a loved one who cares, and in the listening ear of someone who knows what you're going through, all you have to do is look and reach out, and someone will be there to share your troubles."
–Author unknown

After shopping one day, I decided to have a cup of coffee. At the time, my hair was barely growing back following the completion of my chemo treatment, so I was used to the stares and always wore them as a badge of honor. At the coffee shop there was a line of customers ahead of me, but I was in no hurry. The woman in front of me about my age was helping her husband give their order of coffee. While her husband repeated it to the clerk, she glanced back my way. She smiled and to my surprise, she started to chat. She looked directly at me and commented that she liked my "do." I didn't know what she was referring to and smiled hoping that she would explain herself. But then I caught on. She was talking about my hairdo!

She followed her comment with, "Where did you have it done?" I just stared at her wondering if she was kidding me. I answered quietly, "It's due to chemo." She leaned in toward me and questioned loudly, "What? There's a Chemo shop in Red Wing?"

By that time, hearing the conversation, her husband

realized her error and looked perplexed and a little embarrassed. Suddenly her mouth opened wide with awkwardness and sincerely she replied, "I'm so sorry."

I told her it was nothing. As they picked up their order and were about to leave, she touched my shoulder and softly whispered, "I hope you get well." Her kindness brought tears to my eyes.

During a lengthy fight with cancer, there will be countless times of your life where you will need help accompanied with kindness. When a person is diagnosed with cancer, or any other crisis, thoughts become mangled and anxiety can suddenly come upon you.

Questions flood your mind. How will this change in my life; how do I deal with daily responsibilities? Who will take care of the children's needs, my mate's needs, how about my work? You may worry about finances. These needs and many more must be considered first and foremost since whatever affects you and your health will affect your family. When these concerns are dealt with, you'll think clearer and make the necessary choices regarding your care, treatment, and ultimately your healing.

When a friend or relative comes over or calls asking you what can be done for you, don't shrug the request off. Whatever you are presently going through, you need someone now more than ever to assist you in many areas. This is the time to appreciate God working through your relatives and friends, those led by the Lord to be a beneficial factor in your life. Accept their love and kindness. You'll be better off for it, and they will too.

I recall such acts of kindness given in many different ways. I received flowers from loved ones routinely during chemotherapy. Although I dreaded those treatments, I always looked forward to finding flowers waiting for me at home. Another precious gift welcomed me at home in the form of a huge fish tank which was positioned across the room where I rested after chemotherapy. I won't forget how watching those fish swim about relaxed me and renewed my mind and spirit. One friend gave me a CD of an evangelist reading scripture pertaining to healing. Some called or emailed me regularly for an update, and what a treat that was! Knowing that a friend cares and is willing to take the time to see how you are makes all the difference in the world. Others sent get-well cards with meaningful thoughts in their own handwriting. I still have them all. When I was so weak, a dear friend even helped me change the linen on our bed. Our daughter came from Florida for a week to assist with my care, giving me full attention by meeting each need of mine and her dad's too. What a blessing.

Give specifics when others offer to lend a hand. Suggest that you would love some frozen meals to store for the family when you feel too worn out to cook. Include asking for some desserts—cookies for the kids. The dog may need walking, or the children's lunches prepared for school mornings. The yard may need tending to, clothes washed, garbage emptied. Don't be shy in making your requests.

Your mate will need encouragement too. To offer some relief, a friend can plan events with the one who is your regular caregiver to give him a time off, relieving any stress. My husband appreciated talking with another male friend regarding my condition. Several friends met that need in his life during my illness, something I couldn't provide at the time.

I was often fatigued and so if friends came over, I informed them the house may not be cleaned. In my case, my husband was able to take over that chore, but friends never minded how the house looked. One couple brought over an evening meal with all the trimmings and all I had to do was join them at the table. Even at that, I had to excuse myself and retreat to the sofa. You may not feel at your best, but remember people will always understand. Some may feel helpless when you are suffering, but your gratefulness will put them at ease. The scripture says to, ". . . Give thanks in all circumstances, for this is God's will for you in Christ Jesus." (I Thessalonians 5:18)

Advice for Helpers:

Many of you will attempt to put yourself in your sick friend's shoes by trying to do what only they can. Ask the Lord to reveal to you your loved one's needs and do everything with sensitivity to the privacy and emotions of the one who is ill. Would they rather have you come to help out while they are having treatments at the hospital/clinic, or when they are resting at home? Do they need rides to daily radiation treatments? Friends are willing to make a sacrifice in their schedules to help out, so making a working schedule to do errands, or drive for treatments and the like may be an answer to spreading the love of others to the patient. Many sick people are blessed by someone reading Scripture to them, or by watching together a movie comedy, or getting out of the house for a couple hours. Use your talents in helping your friend such as washing their hair, doing their nails, if you are handy at such things. Think of ways you can easily fit into your schedule on how to comfort and encourage your friend. Believe me, whatever you do will be greatly appreciated.

Let's pray together:

Dear Loving Father, I thank you so much for those who love me and are willing to sacrifice their time while they are busy with their own needs. Please bless them with peace and success as they reach out and serve others. Someday, Lord, allow me to return their love. In Jesus' name. Amen.

Chapter Six

How One Can Help by Being Sensitive

"Be devoted to one another in brotherly love. Honor one another above yourselves." **(Romans 12:10)**

Every outreach of empathy with sincerity is appreciated by the ill person. But at times there are those who do not think before speaking. For instance, we who are ill don't want to hear that "things will get better" because such a statement doesn't compute with us. We're suffering *now*, and often times we just can't project into the future as well as we would like to. Other times people will say things like, "So and so is very sick with . . . ." (You fill in the blank.) This is said in the attempt to help the sick person put things into perspective. However, it doesn't work, because some of us may interpret that statement to mean that our illness is less important than another's. To us, our sickness is genuine and we need your full attention. Besides that, thinking of someone else's sickness uses up our stored energy needed for our own healing.

I was often told that I "looked good." But inside I knew I didn't look or feel good. A better greeting is: "How are you tolerating your treatments?" This opens the door for open conversation if the person wants to let you know how they are feeling at the moment. Don't assume we are doing OK by how we look.

One secret that will facilitate communication with a person with cancer is, don't be glib. Don't have the answer to a certain unknown before you find out their story. Listen instead. And while listening, be open to the Holy Spirit's voice prompting you as to how to respond to an ill person's needs.

Each person is different. Some like to talk about their situation as soon as they're diagnosed, others won't. Find out which is which by first listening and observing them. I realize that at times it is helpful to have an answer for those suffering; however, in my experience I found the tenderness of *not* speaking can triumph over unanswerable questions. There is always time to add a comforting word but let it happen at the correct moment.

At times when a person hears of your plight, it immediately reminds them of someone in their family, or a friend, or sadly, themselves who went through cancer. In my case, they eventually would tell me what that particular person did for treatment. These kind-hearted people wanted to make me well—their way.

I received countless suggestions, advice in letters, books, tapes, and the like, which caused my head to spin, so much so that finally my dear friend, Hannelore MacKinney, took upon herself to critique all in-coming mail on my behalf. Her actions greatly blessed me and helped me to concentrate and to act on what treatment my husband and I had agreed upon.

My solution wasn't one I would like as it turned out, but I was led by God and it was the path I would take with His guidance and protection to the point of my complete recovery.

All of us mean well. Since having cancer, and now dealing with lymphedema, I have absent-mindedly said

and done things that were out of line to those now suffering with cancer, or are experiencing some other crisis. If this happens to you also, sincerely correct yourself
and approach the person differently the next time. Think
through what you want to convey in love before seeing,
writing, or calling the person again.

Let's Pray Together:

Dear loving Father, I want to help my friend. Lead
me into expressing my concern adequately to meet the
needs of _____. Use me to convey your love
and peace. Lord, I want to be a help to my friend, not
a hindrance. Guide me accordingly. In Jesus' name.
Amen.

Chapter Seven

Following Your Own Beat from Start to Finish

**"We don't see things as they are;
we see them as we are."
-Author unknown**

Remember the wise advice the young doctor gave me after I was first diagnosed? Each of us vary in nature and with each case of cancer, treatments differ. I had to have surgery, others don't. For example, here I sit; I am grieving at this moment. I have lost a breast. I am feeling sorry for myself. My sister, Alice Peppler, upon hearing me utter these sad thoughts, wrote words to me that lifted me up immediately. She commented, "I'm sure it is hard. God made you another way. God saved you this way. Concentrate on the latter."

The Lord knows my heaviness and sorrow at times, and He knows yours too. My assurance comes from knowing that He is faithful. You may be entirely different in how you respond to a sickness from the person receiving chemotherapy treatments sitting right next to you at a cancer clinic. Stand firm in knowing that your method of recovery is the one chosen for you, and it will make a difference in your life.

Keep going forward with a positive look taking care to glance back ever so often to remember how others helped you through to where you are today. Cancer is part of your past. Put the memories to good use by helping others by what you have learned, by listening to their stories, by praying for them.

We see circumstances from our own point of reference. That's why so many who comfort you will come at it from their personal view point, which often doesn't apply to yours. As a result some with cancer gather with those who similarly have gone through much the same crisis. During my treatments, I attended the monthly luncheons for survivors of cancer. See what your community offers for companionship and learning experiences. Find people who encouraged and answer questions you may have on anything regarding cancer. (Refer to Index for resources.)

When asked, our personal cancer stories can help strengthen and encourage others with the disease. I remember clearly a lovely woman who had cancer of the breast and later lymphedema long before I struggled with either. She and I would meet in passing and asked one another the proverbial question, "How are you?" One day it wasn't enough and we talked in detail how we were progressing. As a result, our experiences broadened each other's. At a certain point of reference, we decided the next time we saw each other and after our chat, we would sincerely state, "Be well!" What a profound difference that made to each of us. We were free to accomplish that direction of healing in our own way. That's very important to allow one suffering to press on to their personal victory, doing it their way—walking to the beat of their own drummer.

Whatever the circumstances, Jesus will see you through. I've learned when dealing with an "unmovable object" such as sickness and pain to simply believe these simple words, "This too shall pass." These four words of truth put things in correct order.

They give a hope which yields to the Lord and His loving mercy, equipping one to carry on even under extreme emotional stress and physical pain.

Bible References:

Here are more Bible references of the blessings that God has for us all through an hour of difficulty. May they strengthen you each new day.

"I consider that our present sufferings are not worth comparing with the glory that will be revealed in us." (Romans 8:18)

"Consider it pure joy, my brothers, whenever you face trials of many kinds, because you know that the testing of your faith develops perseverance. Perseverance must finish its work so that you may be mature and complete, not lacking anything." (James 1:2-4)

"You need to persevere so that when you have done the will of God, you will receive what he has promised." (Hebrews 10:36)

"Those who sow in tears will reap with songs of joy. He who goes out weeping, carrying seed to sow, will return with songs of joy, carrying sheaves with him." (Psalm 126:5-6)

"But we have this treasure in jars of clay to show that this all-surpassing power is from God and not from us. We are hard pressed on every side, but not crushed; perplexed, but not in despair; persecuted, but not abandoned; struck down, but not destroyed. We always carry around in our body the death of Jesus, so that the life of Jesus may also be revealed in our body." (II Corinthians 4:7-10)

". . . call upon me in the day of trouble; I will deliver you, and you will honor me." (Psalm 50:15)

"As he went along, he saw a man blind from birth. His disciples asked him, 'Rabbi, who sinned, this man or his parents, that he was born blind?'"

"Neither this man nor his parents sinned," said Jesus, "but this happened so that the work of God might be displayed in his life." (John 9:1-3)

"Now a man named Lazarus was sick. He was from Bethany, the village of Mary and her sister Martha. This Mary, whose brother Lazarus now lay sick, was the same one who poured perfume on the Lord and wiped his feet with her hair. So the sisters sent word to Jesus, 'Lord, the one you love is sick.'

When he heard this, Jesus said, 'This sickness will not end in death. No, it is for God's glory so that God's Son may be glorified through it.'" (John 11:1-4)

". . . for I know that through your prayers and the

help given by the Spirit of Jesus Christ, what has happened to me will turn out for my deliverance. I eagerly expect and hope that I will in no way be ashamed, but will have sufficient courage so that now as always Christ will be exalted in my body, whether by life nor by death." (Philippians 1:19-20)

Let's pray together:

Dear Father in Heaven,

I thank you for your love and mercy shown me through my time of crisis. I praise you for my on-going healing. I ask you this hour, Lord, to reach out with your love and touch these readers. Bless each with your never-ending reassurance that no matter what happens in their life, you are with them. Show them your loving kindness and mercy as they go through each stage of their illness. Open a door of complete and total healing for them to walk through hand in hand with you, taking them places they never thought possible. Wrap them in your grace and mercy, and shine through each with your love as they follow you in faith.

Father, bless with good health their loved ones who have helped them along their journey. Give each peace that passes all understanding through your Son, Christ Jesus.

May your face shine on everyone who has at one time suffered with the disease of cancer. We are forever in your loving hands. In Jesus' name. Amen.

"I am leaving you with a gift—peace of mind and heart. And the peace I give is a gift the world cannot give. So don't be trouble or afraid."   John 14:27 (NLT)

Index

Your health care team will give you books on your diagnosis and treatment. Here are some extra helps.

WEBSITES:

www.americancancersociety.org.
Offers endless topics regarding cancer. Includes symptoms of breast cancer: The widespread use of mammograms has increased the number of breast cancers found before they cause any symptoms, but some are still missed. The most common sign of breast cancer is a new lump or mass. A lump that is painless, hard and has uneven edges is more likely to be cancer. But some cancers are tender, soft, and rounded. So it's important to have anything unusual checked by a doctor.

Other signs of breast cancer include the following:
Swelling of all or part of the breast
Skin irritation or dimpling
Nipple pain or the nipple turning inward
Redness, scaliness, or thickening of the nipple or breast skin
A nipple discharge other than breast milk
A lump in the underarm area

www.cancertreatmentcenterofamerica.com.
Offers patients information on surgery, radiation therapy

and chemotherapy in combination with complementary medicine therapies, including nutrition therapy, naturopathic medicine, mind-body medicine, and spiritual support.

www.everydayhealth.com
Offers topics on women's health including cancer help.

www.komen.org
Walks you through decisions you'll need to make if diagnosed with breast cancer. Also includes alternative treatments.

www.breastcancer.org.
Answers just about any questions you may have about cancer.

www.y-me.org.
Offers a hotline, guides to local support groups, and more via this National Breast Cancer organization.

www.cancer.og.
(800-4-CANCER) National Cancer Institute Search. Finds clinical trials in database. Also includes an educational section on breast cancer and pregnancy.

www.berfcure.org
(866-FIND-A-CURE) Supplies interesting articles and archived web casts on screening, therapies, and more. In the Breast Cancer Research Foundation is online library of a research-grant-giving group.

www.facingourrisk.org

(866-824-7475) Helps you evaluate your chances of getting breast cancer. Volunteers can refer you to a center for genetic counseling.

www.ibbc.org

(610-654-4567) Living Beyond Breast Cancer. Offers opportunities to swap stories with others on the message board.

www.wcn.org

Covers gynecologic cancers.

www.curesearch.org

Cure Search National Childhood Cancer Foundation and the Children's Oncology Group helps both parents and children with cancer.

www.cleaningforareason.com

Offers free professional nation wide housecleaning services for cancer victims.

BOOKS:

www.booksoncancer covers breast cancer books, lymphedema books, books for children, cancer in general and many more.

Humor After the Tumor by Patty Gelman, 2004, Prometheus Books. Shares lighter moments of the author's treatment.

Breast Cancer Husband by Marc Silver, 2004, Rodale Publishers. Provides helpful tips on coping for any husband whose wife has breast cancer.

How to Prevent and Treat Cancer with Natural Medicine by Michael Murray, M. D., 2002, The Berkley Publishing House.

Beating Cancer with Nutrition by Patrick Quilin, PHD, R.D. CNS, 2001, Nutrition Times Press, Inc.

"**Coping with Cancer**" magazine. Coping, P.O. Box 682268, Franklin, TN 37068-2268. Around $19 yearly subscription.

Publication Information of Ruth Olson Ministries

You may receive the magazine publication, *Gentle Doves*, in your home mailbox by writing: Ruth Olson Ministries, 30090 Hay Crk. Trl., Red Wing, MN 55066. Phone: (651) 388-2206. You may also sign up for the bi-monthly publication at her website:

www.gentledoves.org.

The magazine is designed to supplement daily reading with Christian teaching and tidbits. It includes columns on recipes, profiles of Christians serving the Lord in their daily lives, a pro-life section, a current Bible study, "Family Talks" covering family's activities, a "Trumpet Blast" section shares up-to-date facts on world happenings, and a "Doves on Line" where interesting websites are noted. "In Their Own Words" page includes the reader's own opinions, poems, and personal stories.

On Ruth's website, you can find out more about the magazine, information on her books, *Jesus Loves You This I Know* and *Keep on Walking*, and about Ruth Olson ministries. Ruth is available for speaking and ministering for your church, home or woman's group.

Gentle Doves is supported by tax deductible gifts.